Steven would like to give a most heartfelt curtsy to the infinite wisdom of Katharine Gates and Paul Harrington. And much thanks to Walter and the three hauntingly beautiful Garschagen girls; and to Leslie Barany and Grey Zeien; and to Eggplant, Elephant and she that drips with Pandaliciousness for supplying me with unearthly amounts of companionship and Excedrin™.

Steven Cerio's ABC Book: A Drug Primer

ISBN: 1-889539-07-4

Editors: Katharine Gates and Paul Harrington
Rhymes: Jonny Cecka with Steven Cerio and Katharine Gates
Designer: Andrea Dezsö
This is the second in an ongoing series of alphabet books inspired by *Maurice Vellekoop's ABC Book* (conceived by Maurice Vellekoop, designed by Michael Economy and published by Gates of Heck in 1998.)
The header font, Thickhead, was designed by Scott Ulrich.

Printed in Hong Kong

Published by Gates of Heck, Inc.
15 Harrison Street New York, NY 10013
(212) 343-8878
http://www.heck.com cerio@heck.com

10 9 8 7 6 5 4 3 2 1

BOOKSTORE DISTRIBUTION:
Publisher's Group West (800) 788-3123

NON-BOOKSTORE DISTRIBUTION:
Last Gasp of San Francisco (800) 366-5121

Steven Cerio's

ABC BOOK

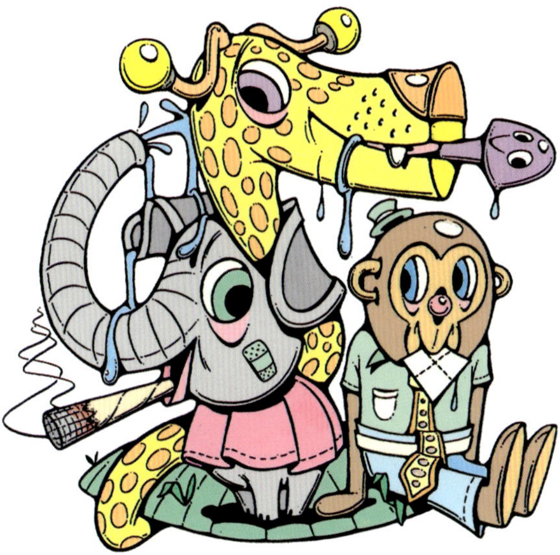

Aa

A is for Angel Dust sprinkled on smokes,
all that you need is a couple of tokes.

Tranquilize elephants or just get them high,
give them enough and they'll think they can fly.

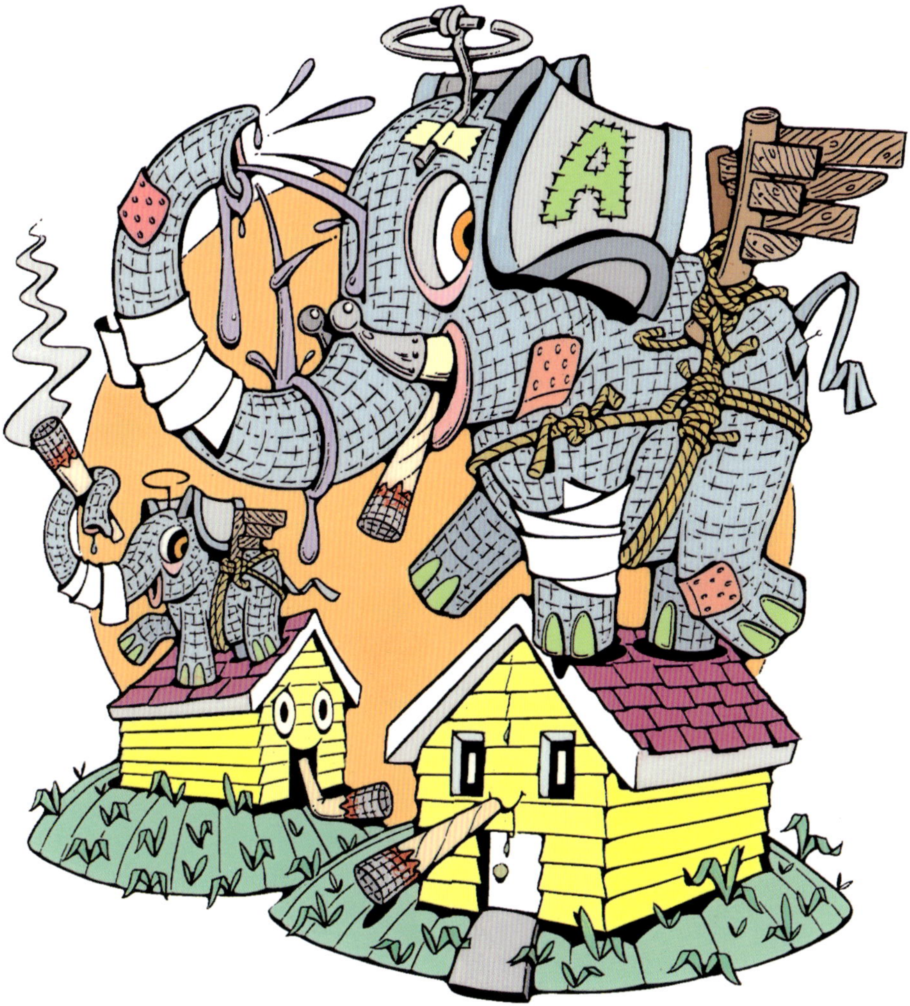

Bufotenine's B, and just between us,
you can get some by licking Bufo Marinus.

Folks come from all over to this unholy nexus,
a town filled with toads in the middle of Texas.

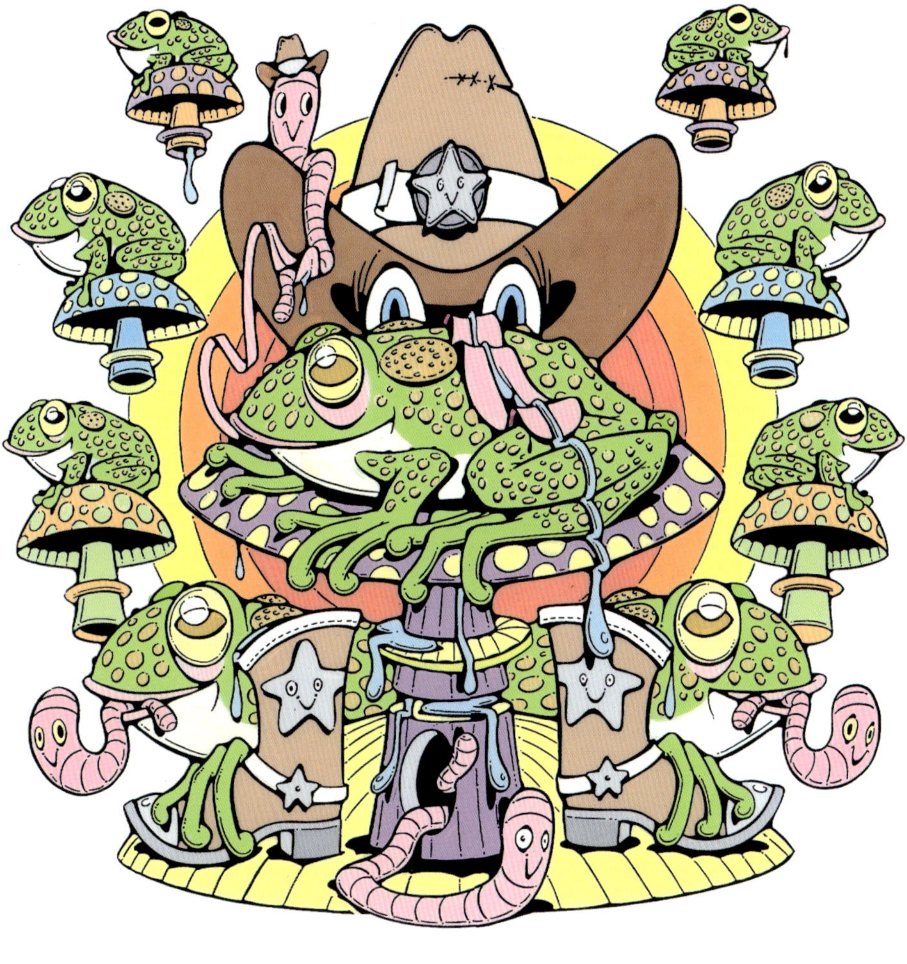

C is for Coke, which you snort up your nostril,

or it could be for Crack, if you like your high hostile.

You can shoot this junk up if you can't stand the wait,

but don't trip this trap, this stuff's powerful bait!

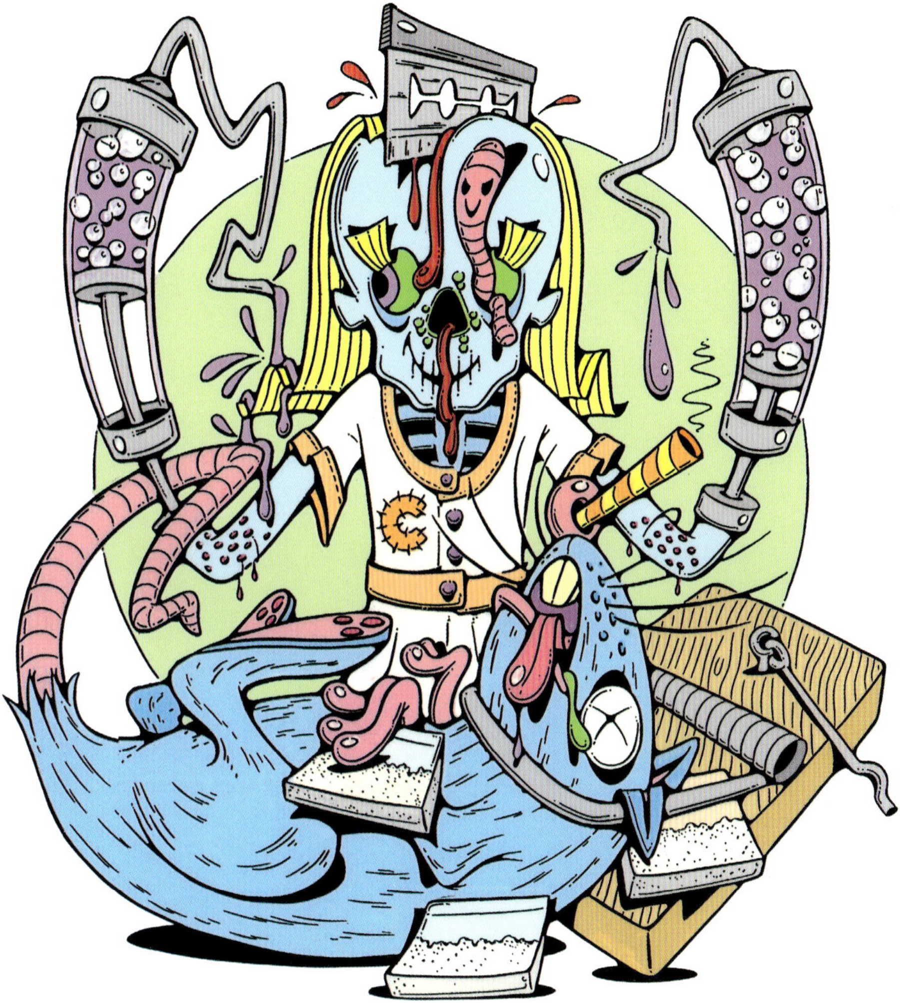

D is for DMT—trips by design,

visit fantastic worlds without leaving your mind.

And don't be alarmed if the pixies torment you,

just tell them that Terence McKenna has sent you!

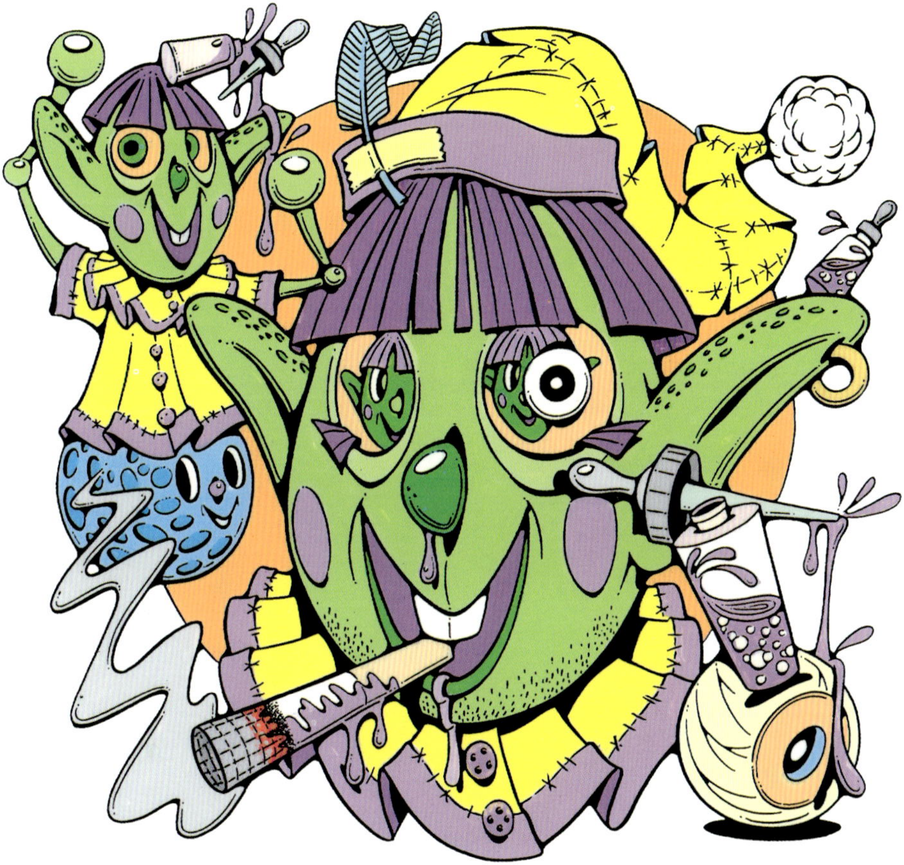

Ee

Ether is E, a Victorian vice,

its heady perfume takes you to paradise.

Meant for doctors to use as a sweet anaesthetic—

Trephination? Amputation? It's all copasetic!

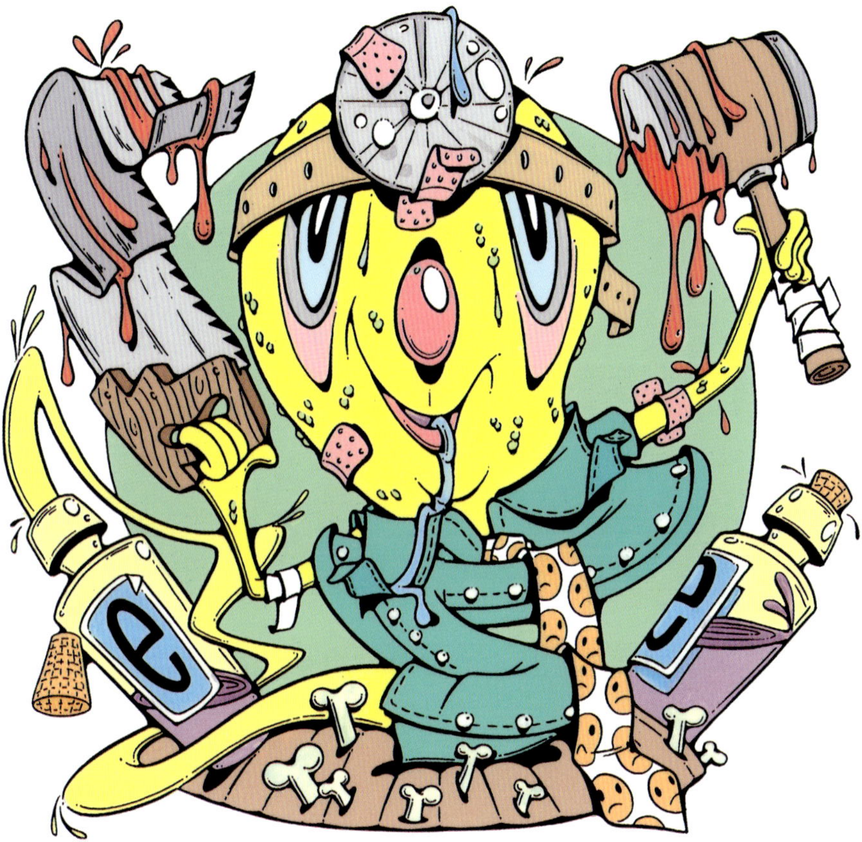

Ff

F is for FenPhen if you think you're fat,
it'll work, so they say, but the problem is that

it causes heart trouble and holes in the brain,
but you already have those if you're truly that vain!

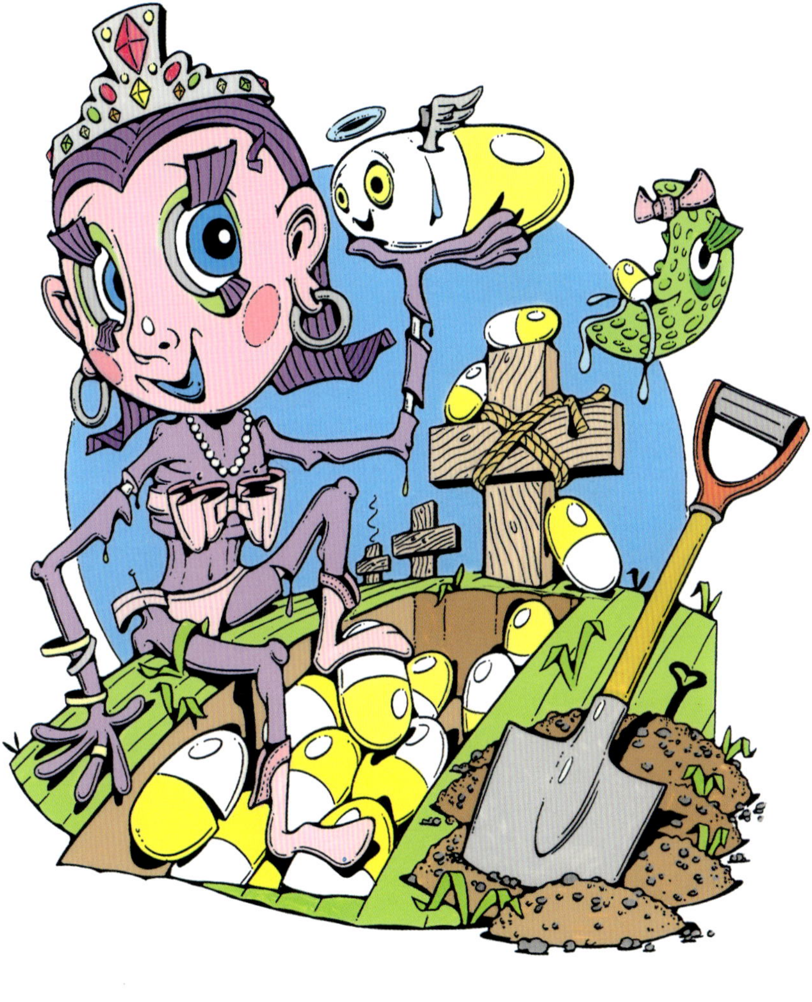

Gg

G is for Grass, some say weed, some say pot,
some use it for "medical reasons"—some not.

Eaten in brownies or rolled in a joint,
You could go get a job, but, hey, what's the point?

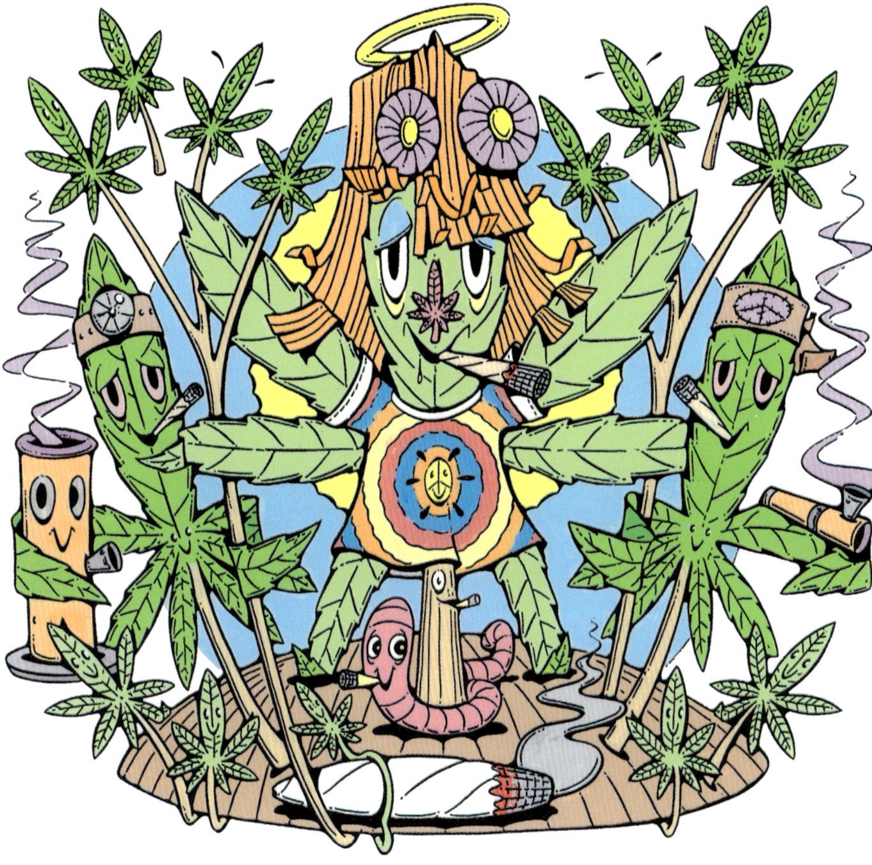

Hh

H is for Heroin, a.k.a. Horse—

but don't ride this pony, unless that's of course

you fancy bad teeth and translucent skin—

you'll go out in style, 'cause heroin chic's "in"!

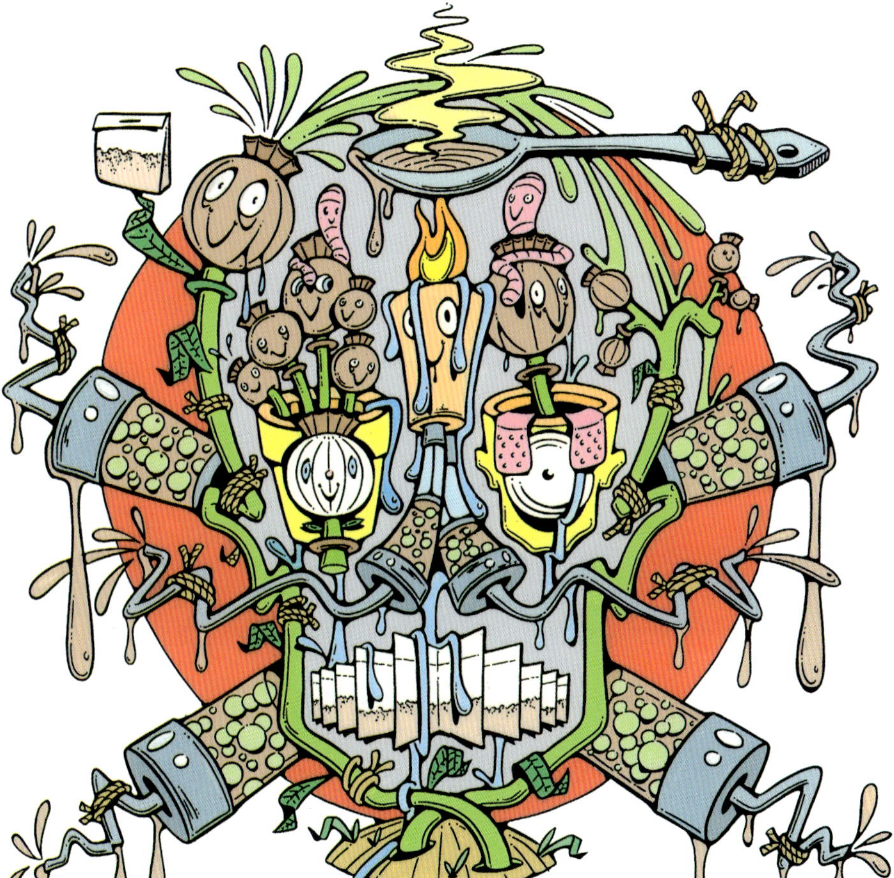

Inhalants are I, and they get you high
by huffing the stuff—here's a few you can try:

Paint and paint thinner, gasoline, glue—
Kids! Kill your brain cells, it's easy to do!

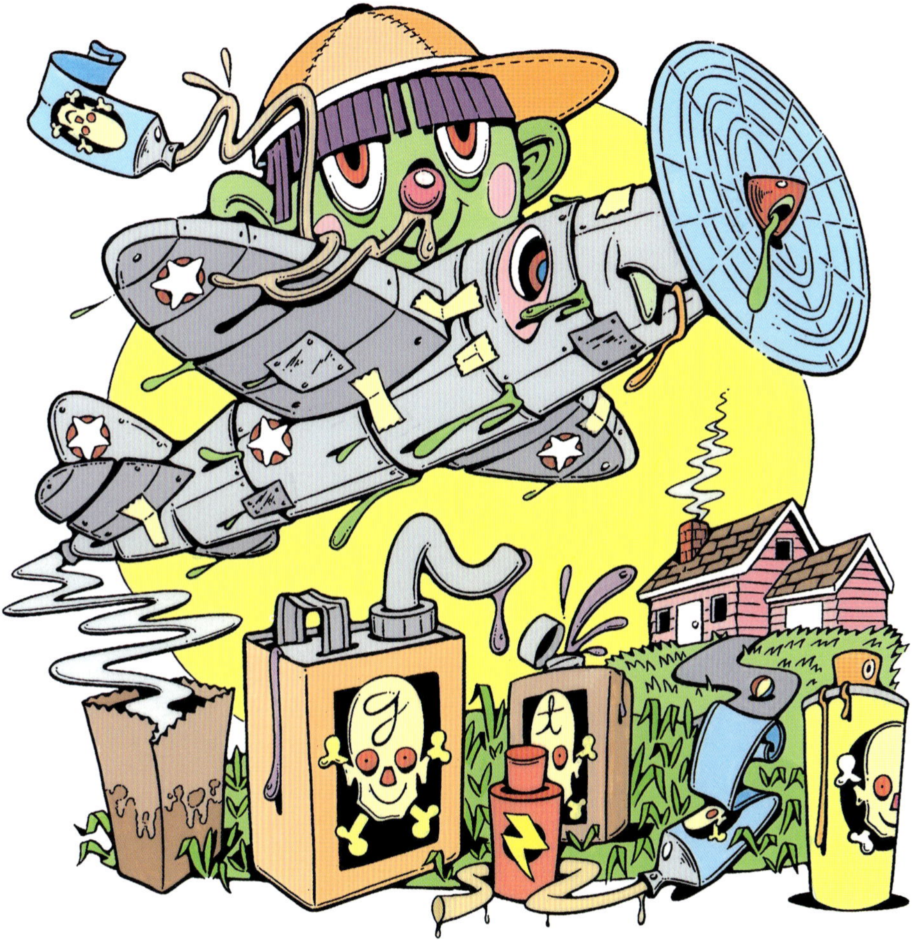

Jj

J is for Java—the drink not the place,

it's packed with caffeine to pick up the pace.

Great with glazed donuts is what most cops think,

Perhaps that's the reason it's still legal to drink!

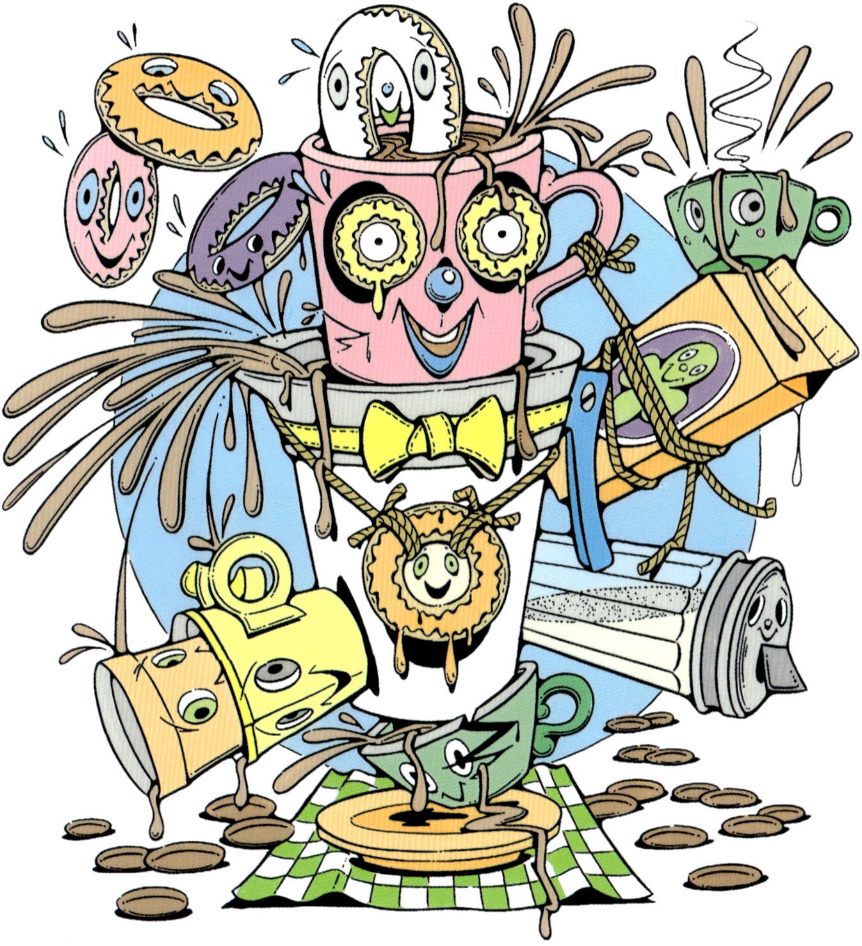

Kk

K is for Ketamine stolen from vets,
Taken by club kids—intended for pets.

Too much Special K, you'll lose motor control—
You'll end up with Alice down Rabbit's K-Hole.

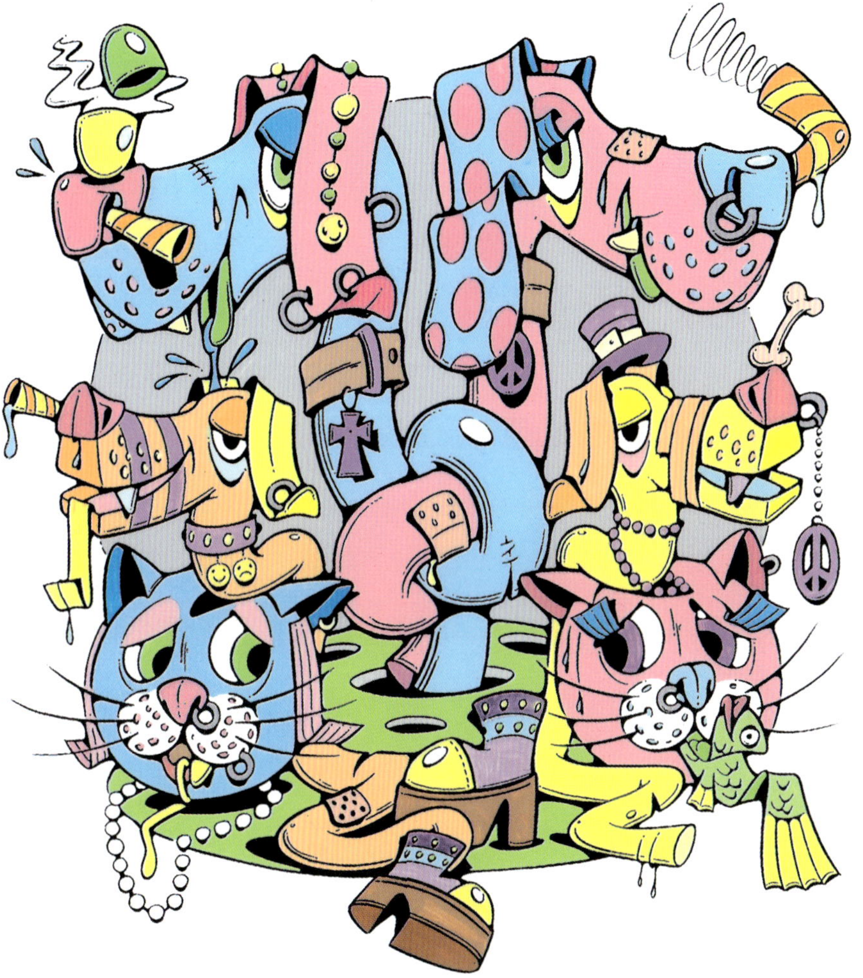

Lysergic Acid Diethylamide's L,

let's just say "LSD" 'cause that's hard to misspell.

In the '60s Tim Leary said blotter was hip,

just a tab on your tongue and have a nice trip!

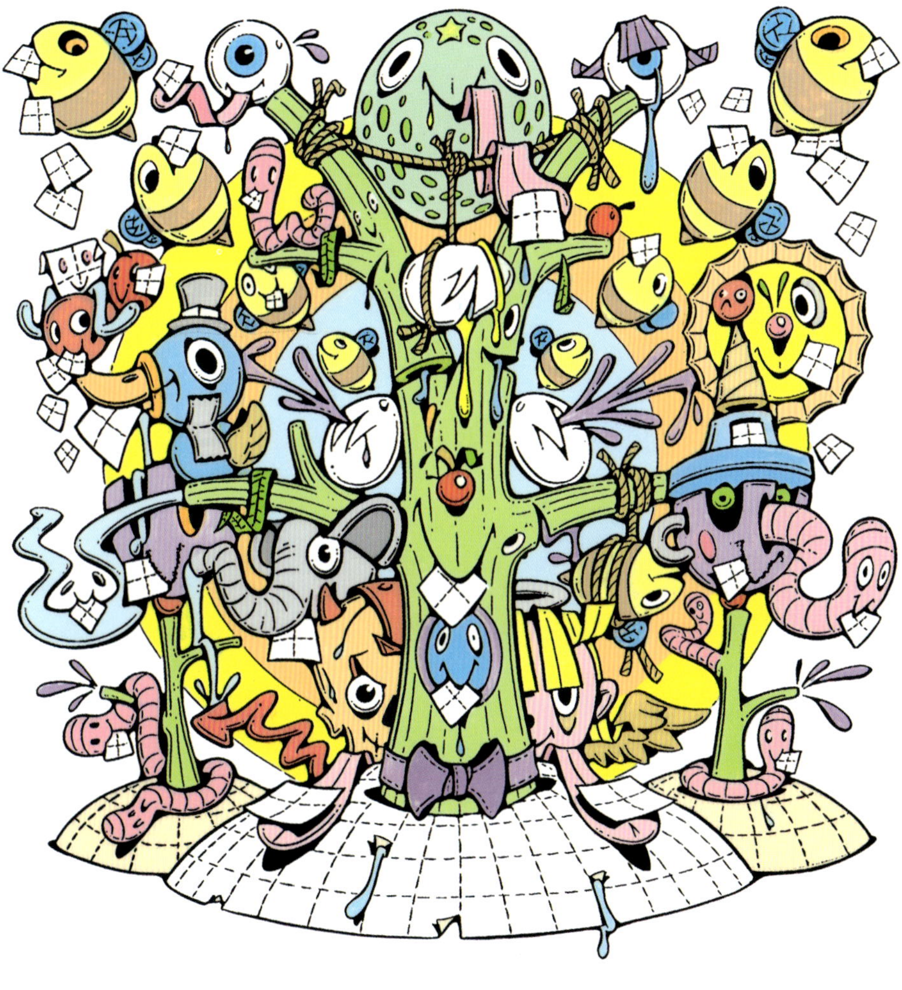

Mm

M is for Methedrine, also called crank,
you'll feel like a shell fired out of a tank.

It's a smash with those hog ridin' bikers and truckers
they make it to sell, to suburban suckers.

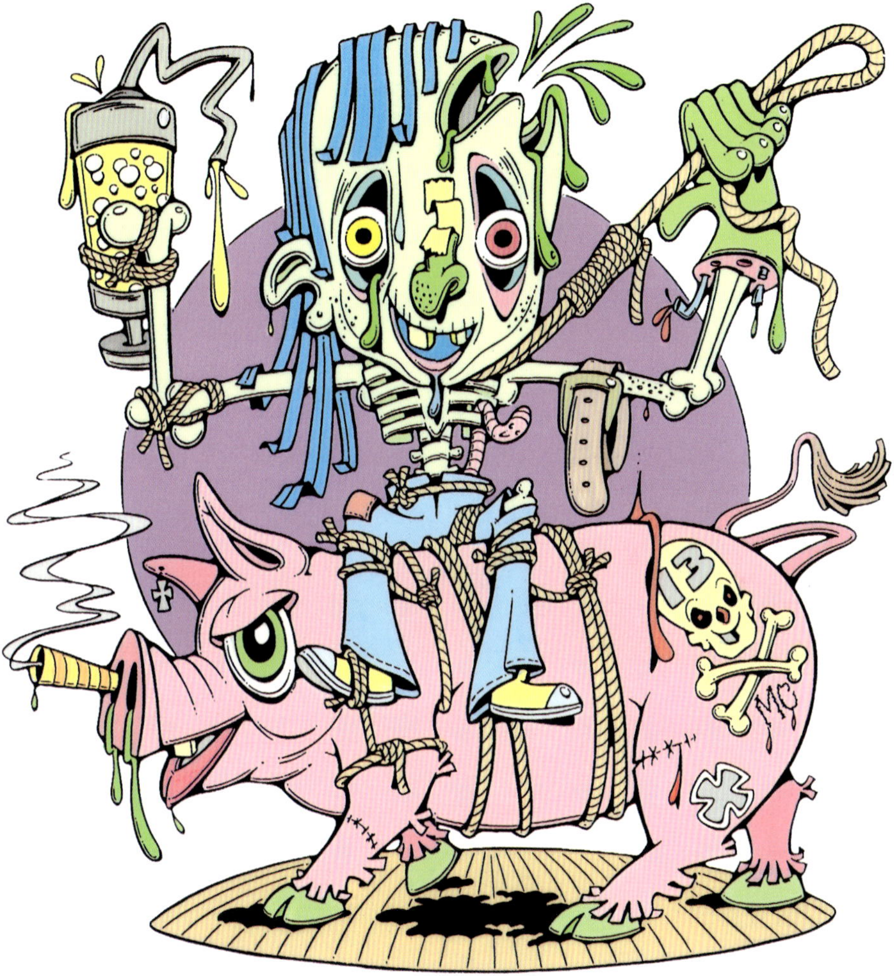
13
MC

Nn

Nicotine's N—it's in cigarettes,
the longer you smoke the harder it gets

to break free of its chains, you're in the industry's thrall,
they claim ignorance but their memos tell all!

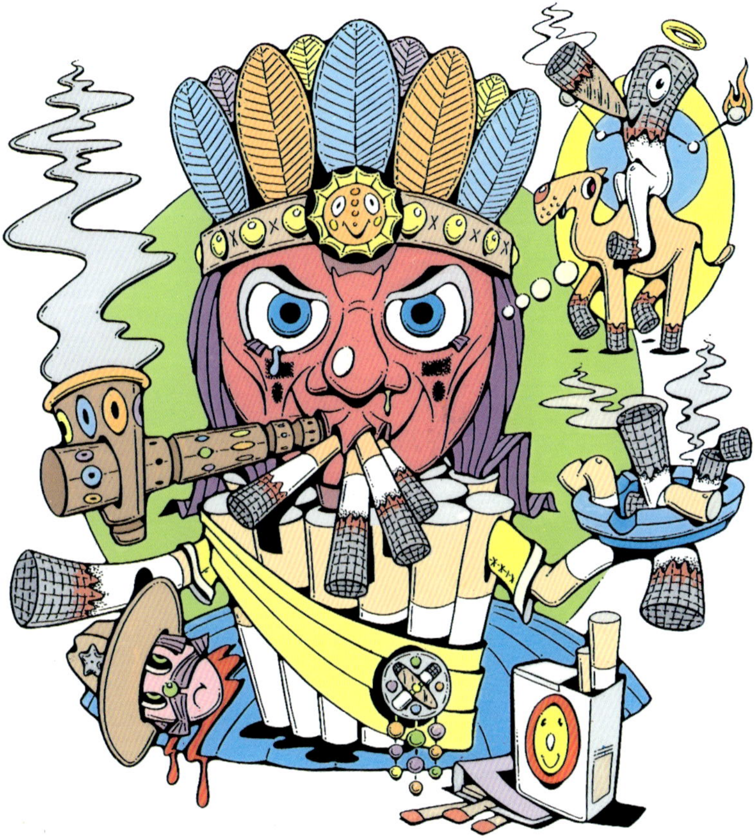

Oo

Opium is O, ‘cause it’s oh so delightful—
the poppy’s your friend but the dragon is frightful.

You eat, drink or smoke it to achieve Zen—
this drug’s so beloved it’s got its own den!

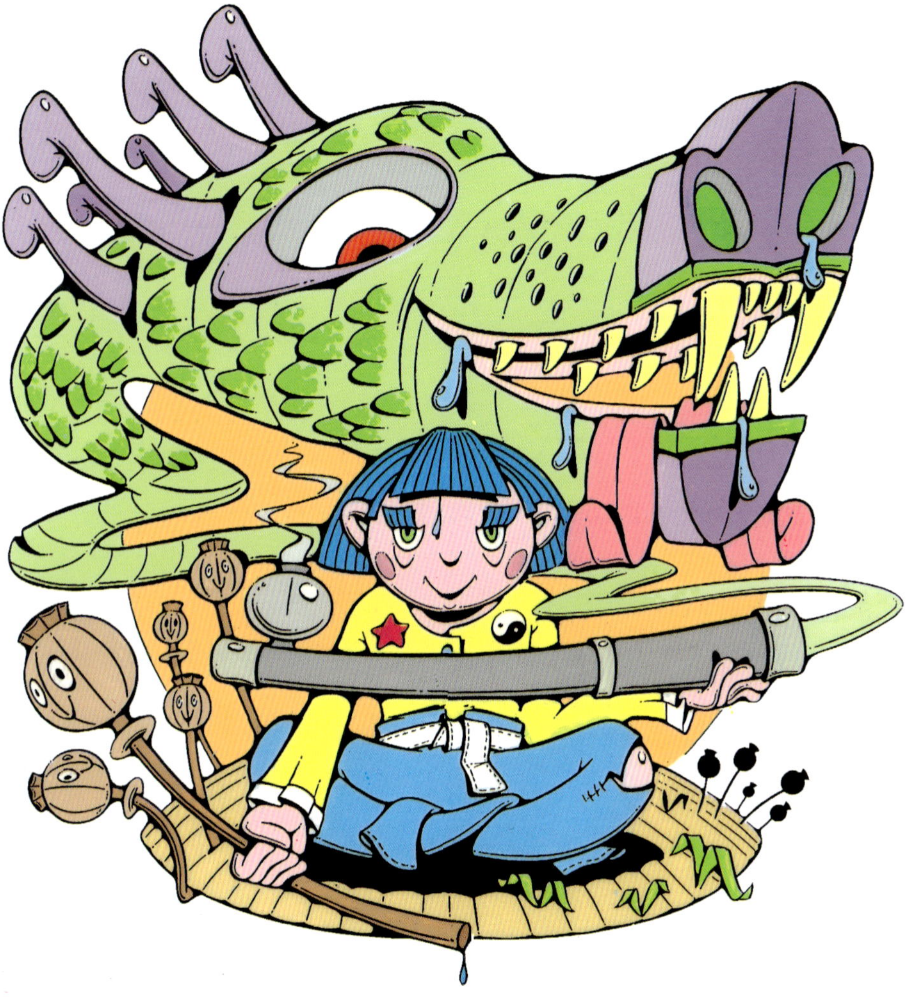

Pp

P is Peyote, that rare cactus flower,
taken by wise men for knowledge and power.

Now hip with the tripsters who chase revelations,
and pasty white hippies with redskin fixations.

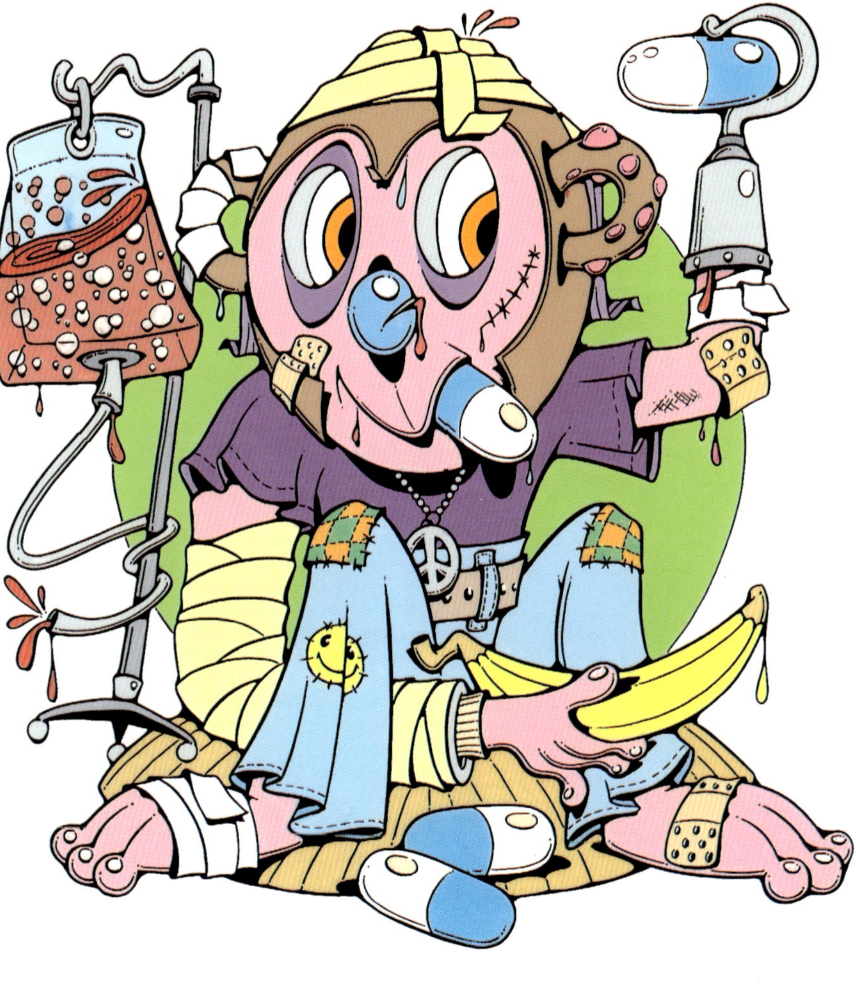

Rr

R is for Roofies a.k.a. Rohypnol,

slip a couple of these in some girl's alcohol.

It dispenses with small talk, you won't have to wait

you can score a home run on the very first date!

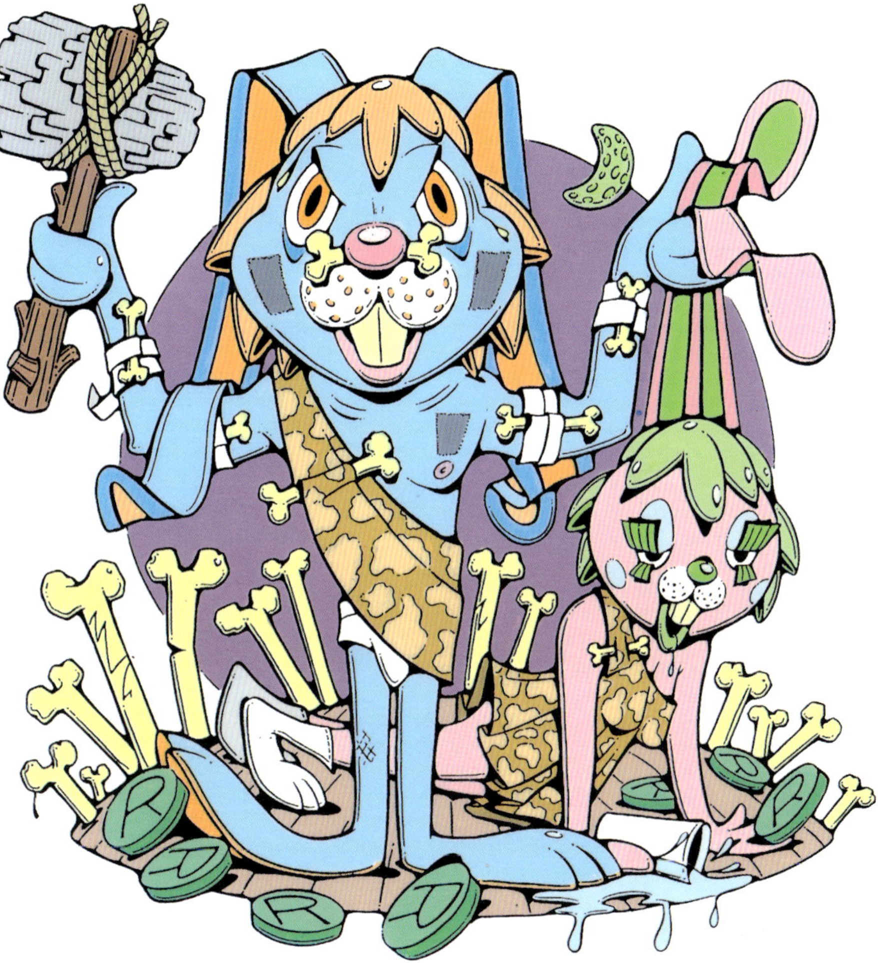

Ss

S stands for 'Shrooms, the mystical fungus,
first sampled by witches and shamans among us.

They must have been brave, to turn coprophagic,
just for a taste of that old black magic.

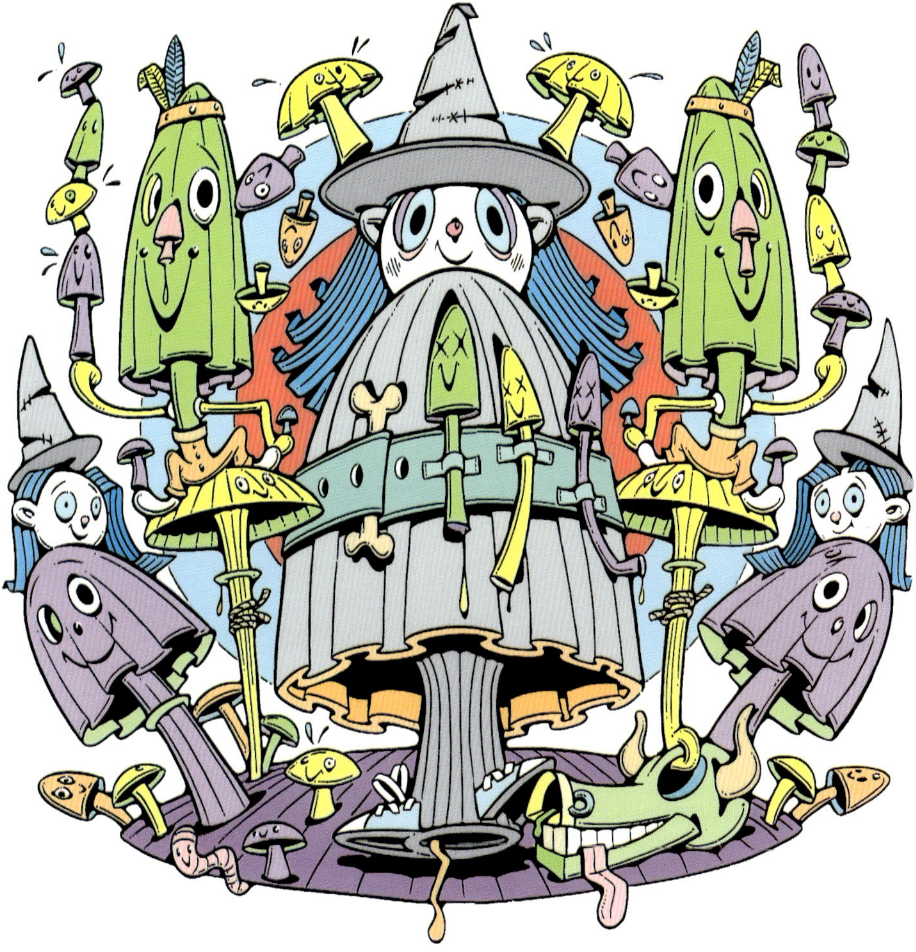

Tt

T is Tequila that Mexican brew,
it messes you up but tastes like an old shoe.

Some salt and a lime will help kill the flavor,
The worm makes you trip, but it's nothing to savor!

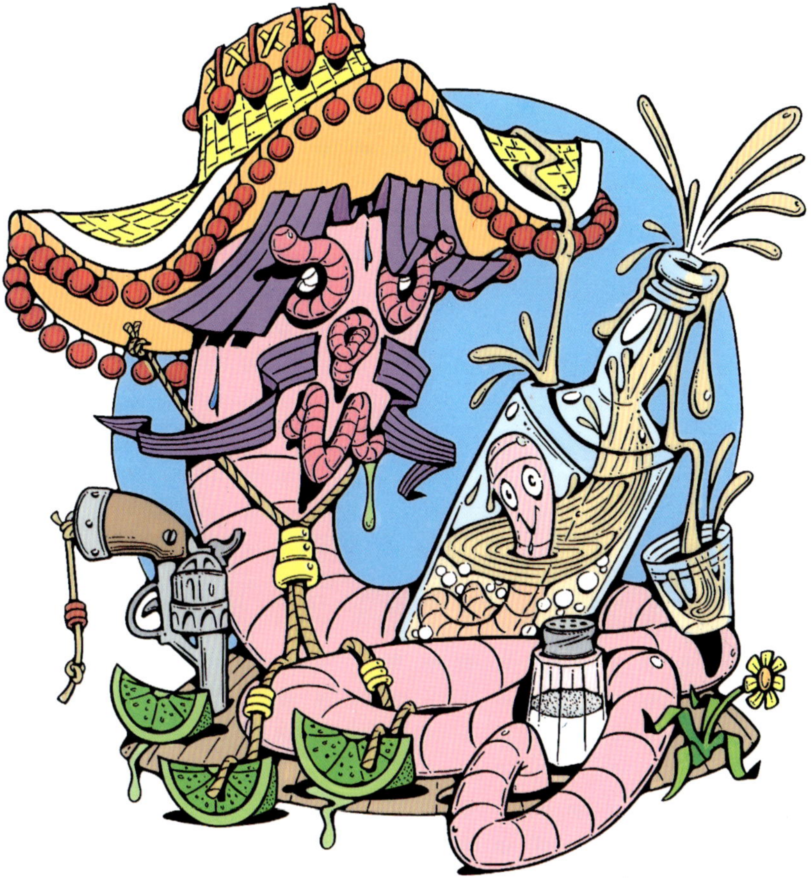

Uu

Uppers are U, a rainbow of pills,

a handful of these and you're amped to the gills.

But beware of what these amphetamines do,

are you chasing the carrot or is it chasing you?

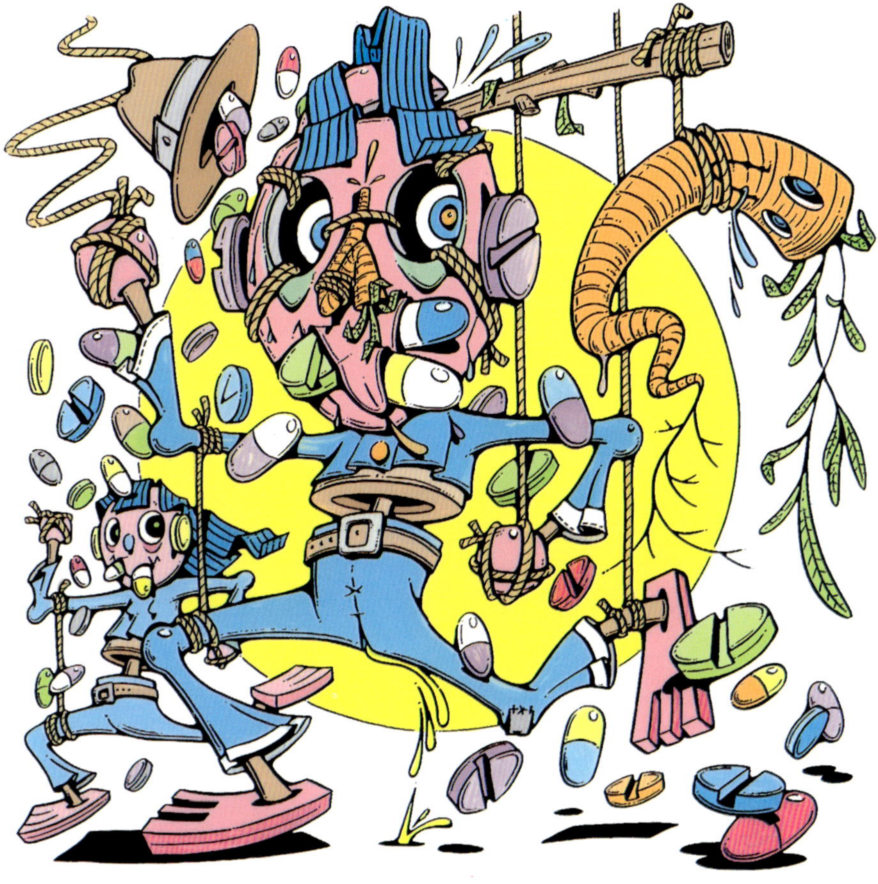

Vv

V is for Valium the famed tranquilizer,
mom's little helper, it helps paralyze her.

She's doing the housework, the kids are at school,
she's clean free of troubles—just watch out for drool.

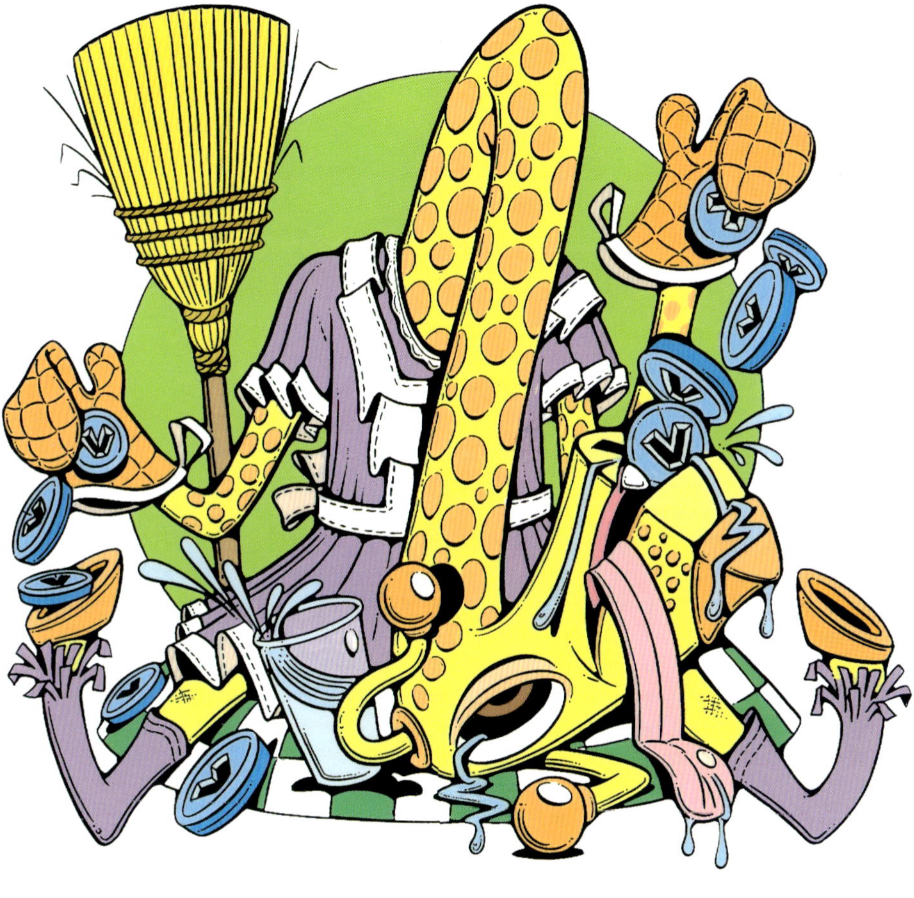

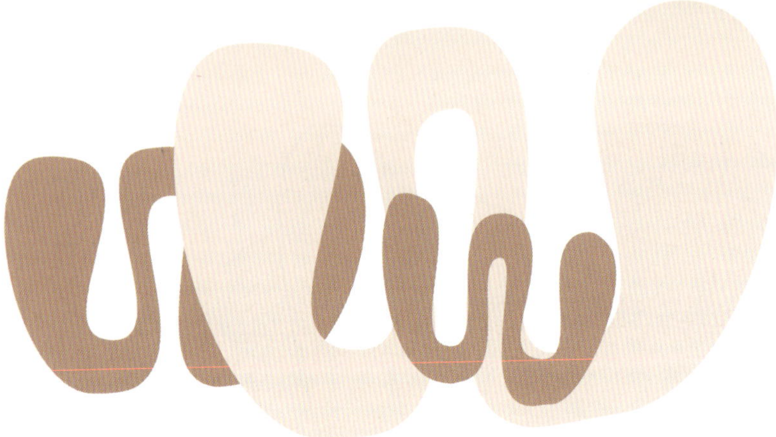

W is Whippets and no, not the mutts,

a few canisters and you're giggling like nuts.

It's for those who like nitrous, intense and extreme,

so let's go to the market and suck some whipped cream!

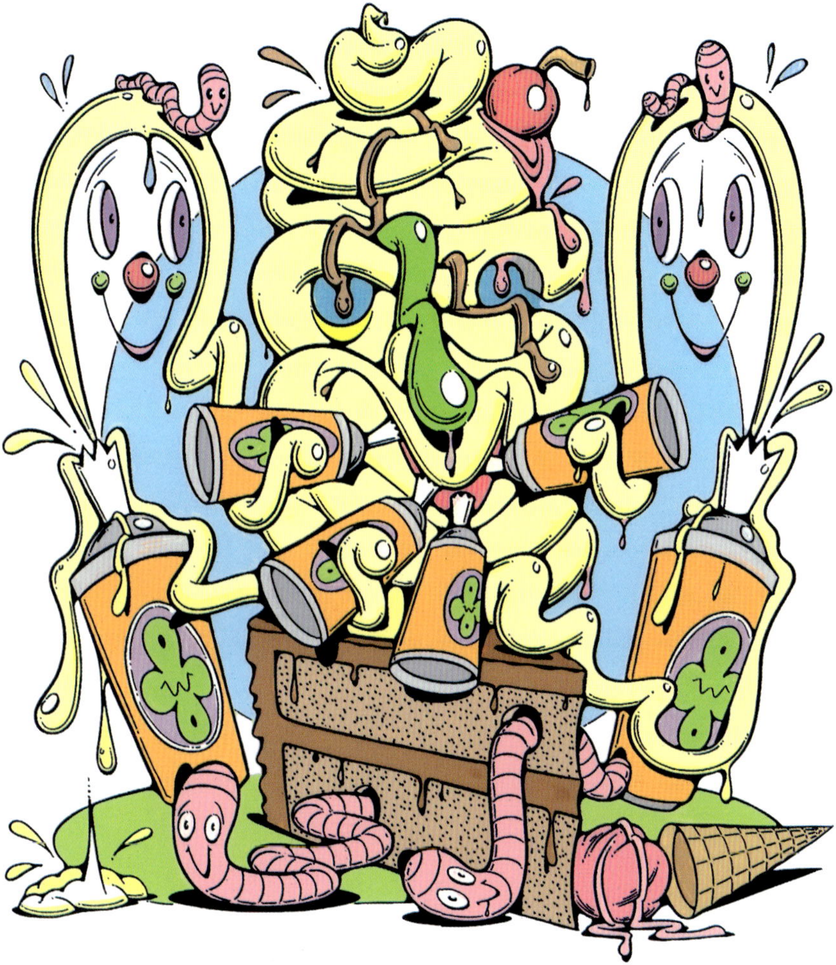

Xx

X is for Xtasy taken by ravers,

and other psychedelic experience cravers.

We shower each other with kisses and hugs,

but it's only because we're all high on drugs!

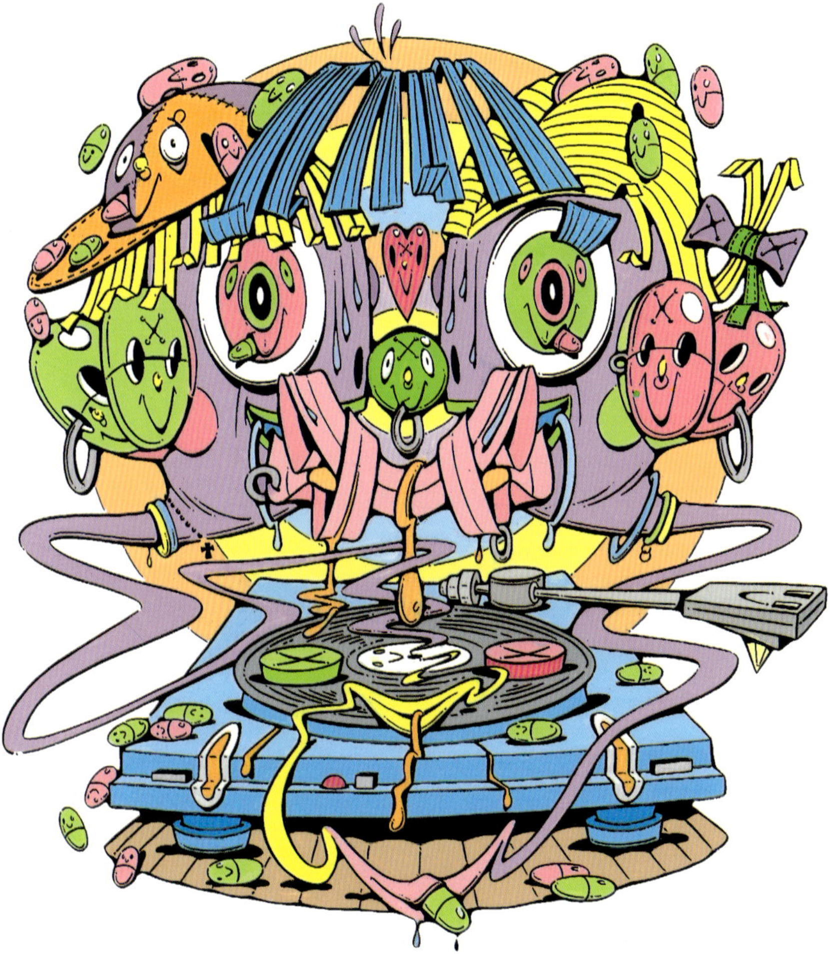

Y is for Yage, food of the Gods,

But beware of Bill Burroughs' big arthropods.

The Great Ayahuasca, Amazonian vine,

imbibe some and become one with the divine.

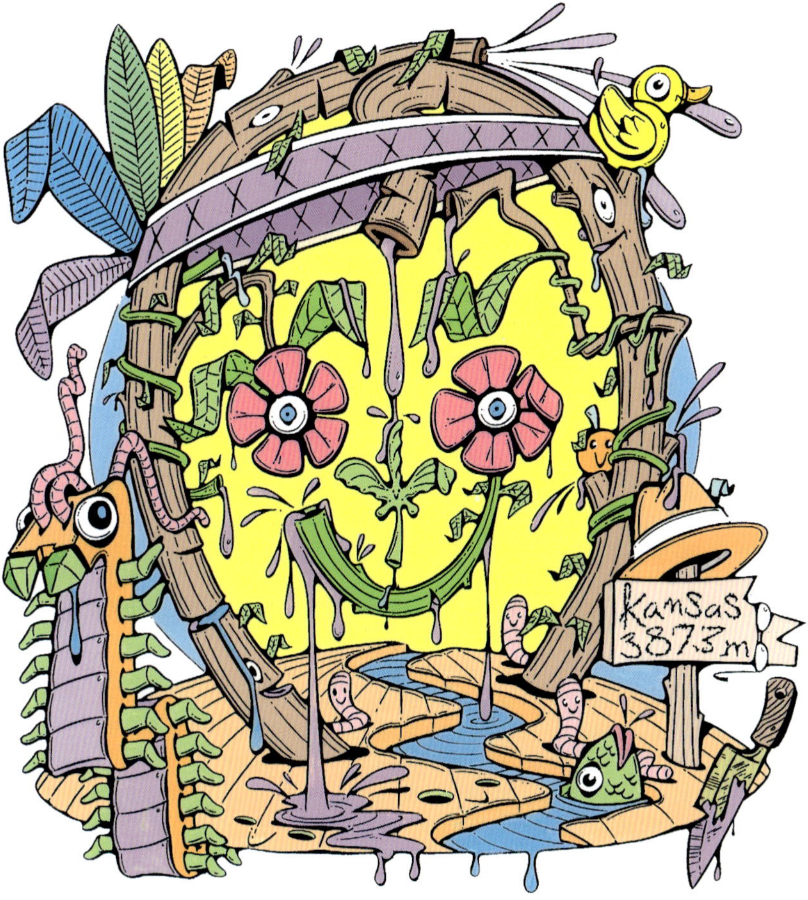
Kansas
387.3 m

Zz

Z is for Zoloft, an SSRI*,
this anti-depressant can take you real high.

It enhances your mood, you're feeling no pain,
you'll float through your tears with a balloon for a brain.

* Selective Serotonin Reuptake Inhibitor

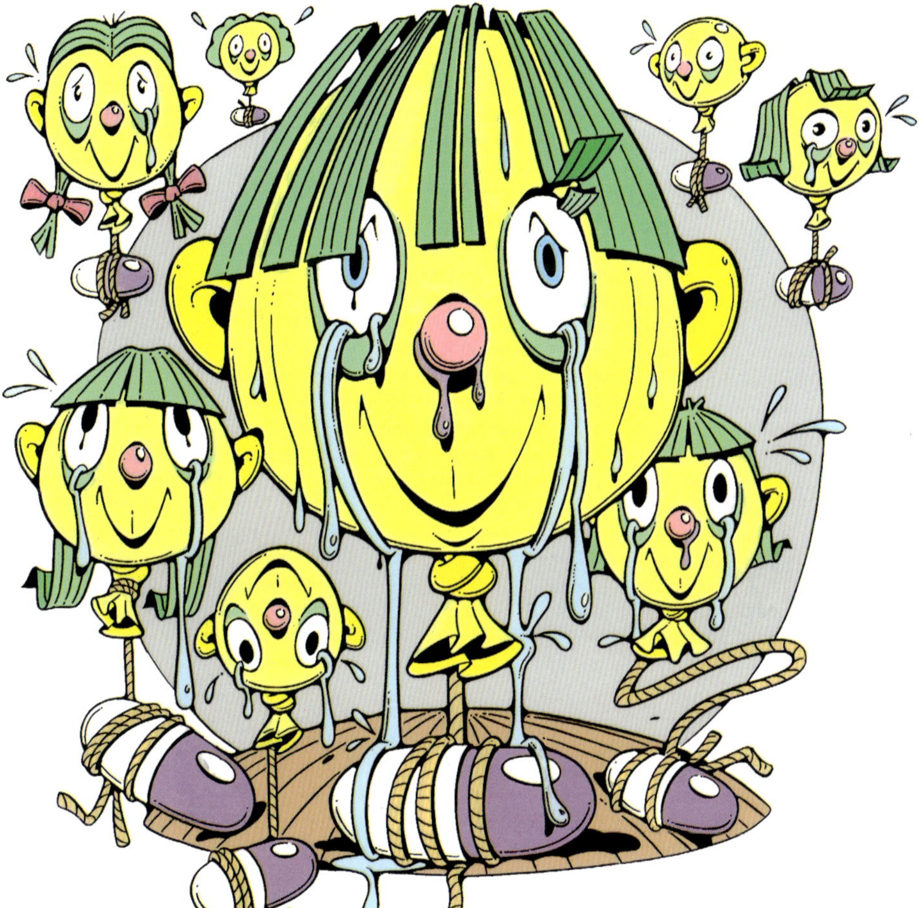

Goodbye boys

Goodbye girls

Goodbye freckles

Goodbye curls

Goodbye hotdog

Goodbye bun

Nice to know we had such fun.

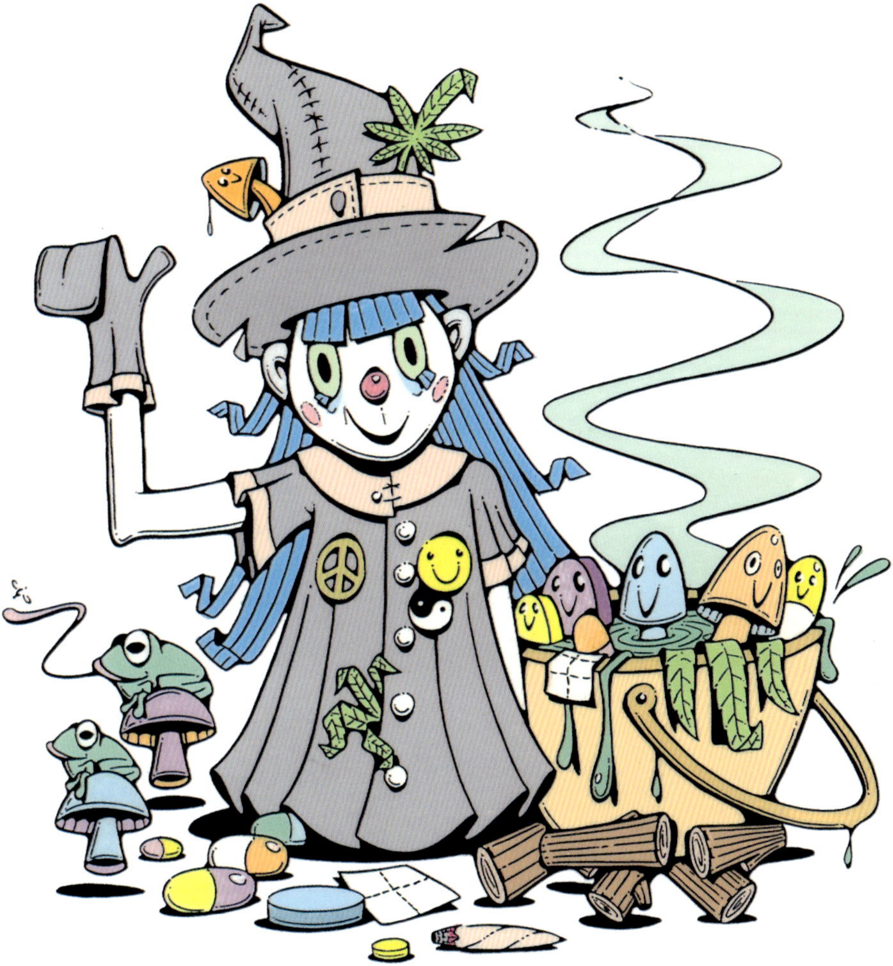

MEET THE ARTIST

Hi, I'm Steven Cerio and I draw and paint a lot; own eleven sets of Tinkertoys™; eat trout every other day; have a purple bike; have been to the world's largest kaleidoscope, world's largest axe and and the world's largest butter sculpture (it was a cow); watch Sailor Moon every Saturday morning; had asparagus for the first time last year and enjoyed it quite a bit; have a friend who painted the inside of his house like an Easter Egg and another friend who refuses to drink water; live next to a mountain; believe that John Coltrane is the one truly great saxophone player; am the Godfather of Luc Sebastian Arsenault; have a scar on my left foot where a snapping turtle bit me and a scar on my forehead where my cousin Tracey hit me with an Etch-a-Sketch™; and I wash my hands before I eat.

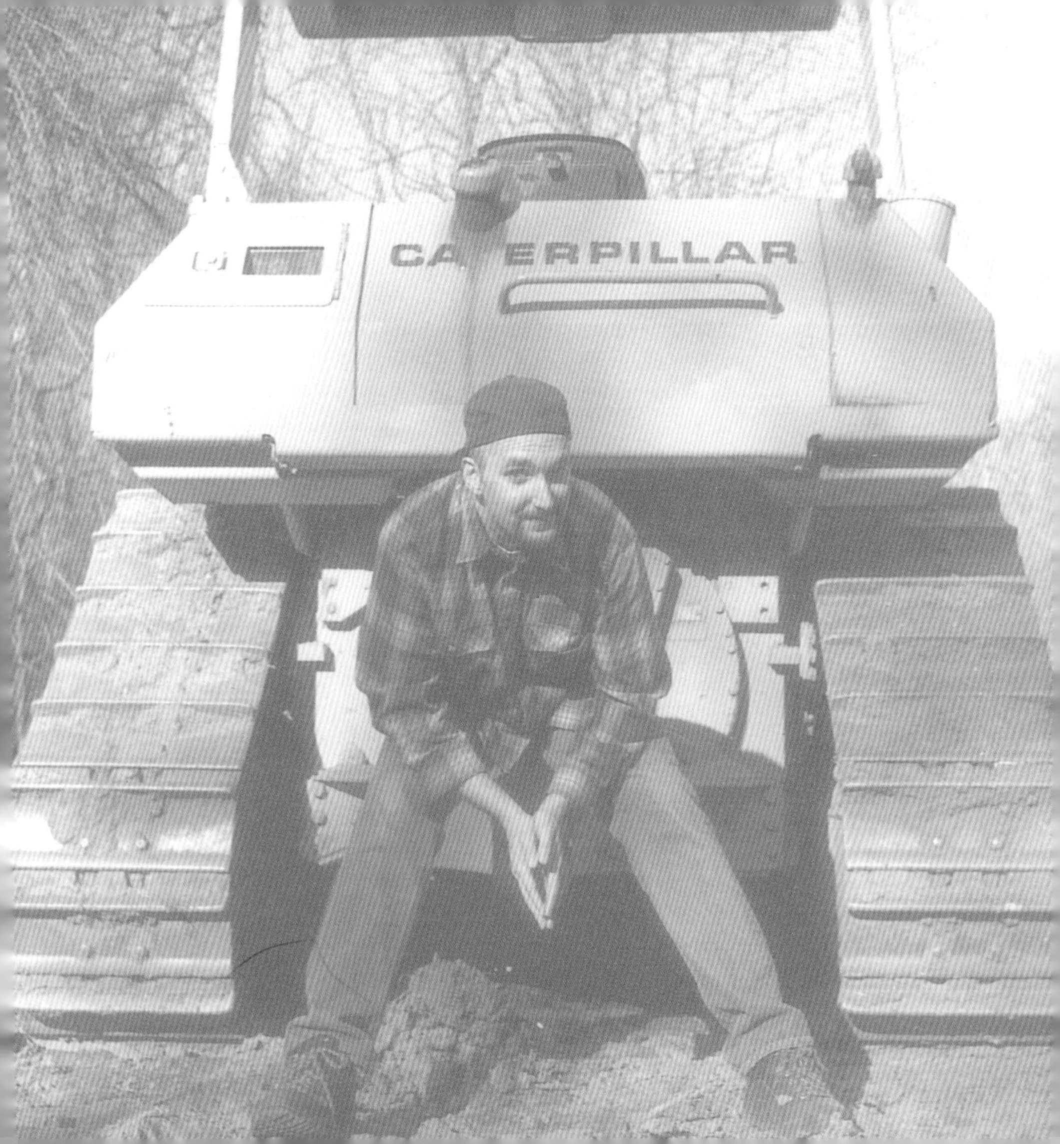
CA ERPILLAR

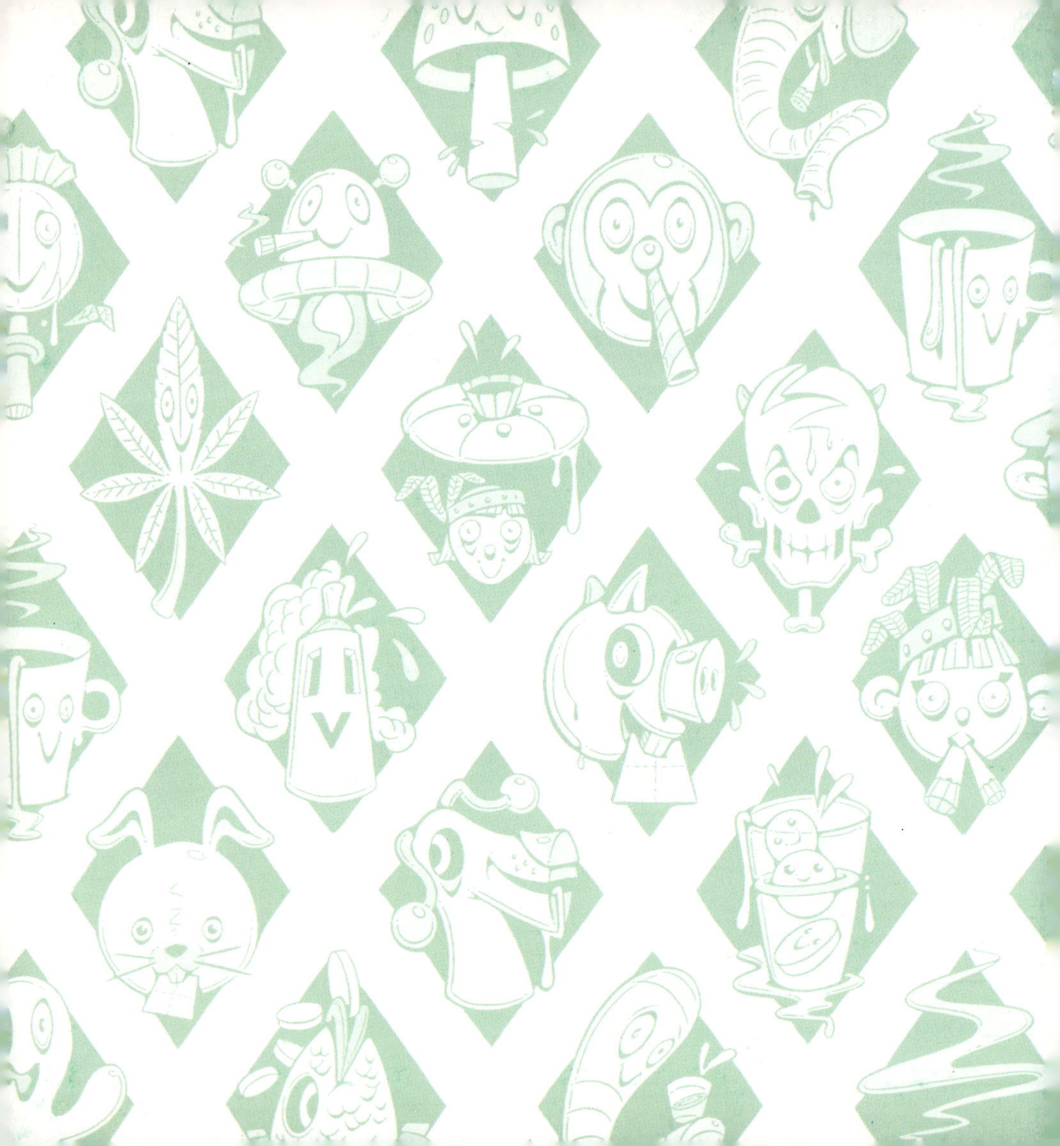